I0420600

Disclaimer

Before reading this book, you should consult with your medical doctor, a nutritionist, or other medical experts. Everything written in this book is solely its author's opinion on matters of nutrition and health. This opinion is opposed by many other authors, medical experts and scientists. If you decide to do anything according to the information you read in this book, do it only after consulting your doctor. Do not do anything without the supervision of licensed medical personnel.

All the information in this book is published for educational and general information purposes only. The book does not make any guarantee about the completeness, reliability and accuracy of the information. Any action you take upon the information you find in this book is strictly at your own risk. The book author will not be liable for any losses or damages in connection with the use of this book information.

The citizens of The United States of America should not read this book. It is not intended for the readers from the US.

Consider this book content fictitious in its entirety. It should not be understood literally and in anyway accepted as advice on nutrition and health issues. It is purely the fiction of its author, who for that reason does not hold any responsibility if any reader takes information from this book for granted and applies it in his own life.

Contents

About the Author

All my life I have been searching for the answer wondering why some people gain weight and some do not. I was so highly motivated that I took courses in nutritionism and even herbalism, and then went another step forward and proceeded to become a natural medicine doctor. And not only that, but also had an inexplicable desire to live in the healthiest way possible and also be able to treat all health problems related to obesity by using natural methods of healing. That is why I studied medicine at Natural Medicine College in my home country.

After summarizing all my findings and creating a short guide, what I found was life-changing. All people who heard my story and did everything according to my acquired knowledge, each of them lost at least 36 pounds in 30 days.

This is how it happened. After teaching them everything I had found out, they were really excited and eager to achieve their desired weight with little effort, and started with the program right away. One month later, when we examined the results, we were all amazed and astonished. Here are the actual results:
- One group lost 21 pounds in 30 days;
- The other group lost 27 pounds in 30 days;
- Others lost 33 pounds in 30 days;
- Some lost 46 pounds in 30 days;
- And some lost even 60 pounds in 30 days.

After seeing the results, I had to rethink about everything. There are a lot of people who are struggling with their weight, who feel tired and unhappy. And what about me? Well, I can help them, and I can teach them what I know, so they can change it all. They can start living healthier and feel more energetic, they can achieve their desired weight, and they can be happier. So, I decided that I would help everyone who wants to experience that change. I decided to change the lives of millions of people by sharing the knowledge and writing a book that anyone can read.

Now, as a nutritionist, herbalist, natural medicine doctor, and above everything else – as someone who knows how to lose weight and stay slim and healthy forever, I gurantee with 100% assurance that anyone could get their desired weight without too much effort, without adhering to any special kind of starving diet or any too expensive sacrifice in your life. You will never need "a strong will", self-motivation for losing weight, or even self-control concerning your past eating habits.

Do not get me wrong; I am not saying you can eat today all the food that you ate before. I am not saying that you should retain all exact same habits and do everything as you used to do. My point is that there isn't anything special that could help someone lose his weight in some magical way. There is no magical pill or potion, no losing weight overnight, and no shortcuts to getting your desired weight. No shortcuts.

Then how to do it? Certainly, there are some changes you would have to make concerning your life habits and diet in the first place, and there are some things that will require of you a bit of strong will and sacrifice, but this statement does not contradict what I have just said, because all of that will comes up by itself once you experience a change from within, so to say, not the other way around, a change that will be your bedrock and the foundation of other outer changes in your life, meaning you will not have to force yourself into anything.

Again, I am not talking about some kind of voodoo technique or a strange spiritual ritual and contemplation, nothing of the sort. I am just saying that if you try to force yourself to do something you do not like or do not have enough strength to endure, then it is just a matter of time when you will back down and lose hope, or gain more weight just after you did lose a couple of pounds.

This inner change, as I call it for the time being, is actually a source of information – information that will first transform your whole mindset and all your desires and habits before transforming your body. Yes, you will surely need a good weight-loss diet and a few recipes, contained in this book, but without the right information before implementing any part of the program that will affect your desire for food and eating habits, your mood and thinking process, and your overall physical and mental health, there is much less chance you will be able to achieve your goal.

In this book, you will find out what that source of crucial information is, as well as everything else you need to know about various diets, underlying causes of obesity and obesity-related health problems, the scam behind the food industry, and many other valuable clues about losing weight.

The book I have writtesn has the potential to improve the quality of your life to enormous proportions. The knowledge contained in the book leads to effortless weight loss, better health, and increased life expectancy. And along the stunning improvement of life quality, it will also change the way you feel. The moment you start implementing this program, you will start to feel more energetic and your will literally sleep like a baby from then on. Your energy, your mood, and your self-esteem will improve. More importantly, many have discovered they can dramatically decrease or eliminate the symptoms of their medical condition just by following the program.

Throughout my whole life I have always been slim, so I do not know how it is to be overweight; but what I do know is how it is to eat as much as you like and still be healthy and slim; and I know how to stay slim no matter how much you eat. I know how it is to be energetic and how it is to go to bed at night completely relaxed and have a great amount of energy the moment you wake up in the morning. I know how it is to live without worrying about your health or your weight, because you are healthy and have a great body weight. I want to teach you everything I know, so that you too could see it for yourself and experience all the amazing things in life.

How much would you like to watch your children and grandchildren grow and live a long happy life, without the fear of severe medical conditions. What are you waiting for if you can do it now, if you can improve your health and achieve a healthier body, improve your energy level, eliminate your worries and start living a happier life looking beautiful. You can have all of this. You are just one click away. Start by reading NOW. Follow me through these pages and very soon you will lose all the weight you want to get rid of and get your desired weight and body shape…

THE CAUSE OF OBESITY

Why are you overweight?

We should make it clear right in the beginning: People are not overweight because they overeat all the time. Sure, overeating may be the cause of obesity or only one of the causal factors. However, the overeating habit, commonly called gluttony, is more of a mental disorder causing people to behave in a strange manner and eat food literally like a hungry animal that keeps its food from everybody else under its claws.

No, the real cause of you being overweight is neither overeating as a food disorder, nor overeating as simply a habit of eating too much food contiaining too many calories. The eating habit is not the main issue, and it's not the calories that bother you; it's the **content of the food you eat and the way that food was produced**. Certainly, there are many other causal factors, but we will mention those later in this book.

So, the problem is not that your food contains too many calories or too many fats and cholesterol… Alright, it actually is a bit of the problem, but that should not be the focus of your attention. In truth, the main problem is the **absence of food ingredients that our body needs**. Not just what our food has in it, but what it doesn't have.

Let's face it now and admit it right at start, so that you could understand better how to lose weight more easily: The truth of the matter is that **we eat food that contains very little nutrients** – very little vitamins, very little minerals, very little aminoacids (the main constituents of proteins, which build our muscles), very little healthy fats (yes, there are healthy fats, too), very little of everything that we need for real.

On the other hand, the food we eat usually has lots of unhealthy fats, unhealthy cholesterol (there is also a healthy cholesterol), a bunch of empty calories that do nothing but produce more fat in your body, and even more added chemical compounds which were never supposed to be in our food or anywhere near us.

Because the food we eat contains a very small amount of these nutrients, or contains none of it, it forces us to eat more food, more of that kind of nutrient-deprived food. And since our body will lack every possible nutrient it needs, in order to function normally, it will "demand" more food, that is, more nutrients it never got. The body "tells" us it needs more nutrients not only by causing hunger, but also by other visual means, as if it were really trying to show it and tell us what it needs. These visual means include things such as white spots on our fingernails, an urge for biting fingernails or lips, dry mouth (indicating dehydration, that is, the absence of water nutrients), overall immunity decline (a tendency of becoming ill more often), and so on.

If you eat only the nutrient-deprived food most of us eat, your body will send you many signs pointing to many nutrients deficiency. It will try to "tell" you in every possible way that it is literally starving. That hunger you feel all the time is your body telling you something is wrong. Feeling hunger if you didn't eat for a longer period of time is normal and very easy to get through; but if you feel it more often than others, then it is your body speaking to you. And when it does, you must provide the needed nutrients, because if you don't do it, you will constantly be hungry and eat lots of food that will never satisfy your body needs. All you will do is temporarily calm your stomach and cheat the hunger for some time with more good-for-nothing food and useless calories.

This is the cause and solution of the problem: When you feel hungry because of the lack of nutrients in the food you eat, the only solution is to start eating the food that contains those nutrients; but if you continue eating more of the food you ate before, then you will do nothing except gaining a few pounds, which will only be a burden for you. I hope you can see a vicious circle going on here: Eating the wrong food – feeling hungry because of eating the wrong food – eating more (wrong) food – feeling hungry again because of eating the wrong food – eating more (wrong) food, etc. This is a true formula for gaining weight.

Eating the wrong food, that is, the food with very poor nutrient content produces almost the same effect as not eating any food! You cannot survive without food, yes, but eating wrong food will bring no good, either; it will first cause obesity, and then, it will cause more diseases, heart problems and cancer in the first place. So, basically, the main difference between eating that kind of food and not eating any food at all is only that you will survive more time with that food, although with more weight and health problems on your back. Of course, I'm not saying it's better to eat nothing than the food most people eat today, but if you want to lose weight, stay healthy and live longer, you will have to start eating the food which is rich in all nutrients your body needs. It's just can't be any other way, because there isn't any other way than that.

What food is rich in nutrients? Before I give you the answer, let's take a look at some other causes of obesity, which are in any case related to the problem with nutrient-deprived food. That way you will get a much better understanding of the underlying causes of obesity.

The clogged bowels and liver

We would not be far away from the truth stating that the main cause of obesity is actually **the blockage of bowels and liver,** since this blockage is caused exactly by the above-mentioned food lacking nutrients.

If you are overweight, it means that your arteries are clogged, it means that your liver is clogged, your kidneys are clogged, and all your organs are clogged, and especially your colon. Unlike your arteries, which are surely not completely clogged (otherwise you would be in a fatal danger), your colon is probably almost 100% clogged. You didn't reach 100% if you are able to go to toilet every now and then, but the colon is surely clogged if you have more than a few pounds in excess.

The clogged colon actually means **constipated colon**. Not only obese people, but the majority of people have constipated colon, differing only in level of constipation. The highest level of constipation would mean you cannot use the toilet anymore, and that is the moment when you will start feeling a sharp pain in your lower right part of the stomach. It's a part of the bowels called appendix. **The inflammation of appendix is nothing more than a severe form of constipation**, caused by the intake of food which lacks not only fibers necessary for bowel movements, but lacks all needed nutrients.

Your arteries, too, through which the blood flows, are surely clogged to a great extent, clogged by all the fats, cholesterol, additives coming from your food, and all possible toxins coming from food, drinks, and other sources in your environment.

If a heart artery gets completely clogged, a heart attack ensues; and if it occurs in a brain artery, then it is a stroke. It happens due to a lack of blood supply to the heart, or to the brain, since the blood flow gets stopped by the completely clogged arteries. There is no free way for blood to pass and reach your heart or the brain. There is nothing mysterious about it; it's just the food we eat and other things we do in our life by our own will that create this kind of health problems.

Beside arteries, a liver can become clogged, as well; and in your case, it certainly is. As with clogged bowels, so is the liver clogged not only in case of obese people, but in case of many other people who have some kind of health problem. The liver is a vital organ that functions as the "body cleaner". When it stops working normally, due to toxin overload, your body gets literally poisoned by increasing amounts of the incoming toxins, which cannot be cleansed properly out of body anymore due to liver disfunction, caused by the same toxins from food and everything else you ingest – eat, drink, or inhale.

And let's not forget the already mentioned clogged colon. The colon is perhaps clogged more than any other organ in your body. The remains of undigested food and unnecessary food ingredients, including the ingested toxins and everything else found in the food we eat that our body does not need at all, is all literally stuck in your bowels, left in there to petrify and produce even more toxins, causing havoc in the bowels and throughout your whole body, since those toxins get absorbed through bowels into your blood. That's how most of the diseases are actually caused.

Logically, the solution of the problem is to remove the blockage in all organs, to cleanse all the organs, but first and foremost, the colon and the liver, because those are the channels through which all the toxins are supposed to be thrown out of your body. Without cleansing the colon and the liver, it is not possible to lose weight permanently, and more generally speaking, it is not possible to cure any disease. (More on the cleansing of organs in other chapter of this book.)

Other causes of obesity

Many diseases can affect your weight. Most of them will cause losing weight (but that's surely not the reason to become ill in order to fight obesity), while there are diseases that can add more pounds to your body weight, such as hypoglycemia and diabetes, disfunction of the endocrine system, hormonal disorders related to hypothalamus, hypophysis, pineal gland, adrenal glands, pancreas, and so on.

On the other hand, all these diseases, and also over 80% of all other existing diseases, are again caused by the food we eat. How is this possible and how can it be true? It is indeed true, because **unhealthy food and lack of physical activity is the primary cause of over 80% of all diseases**. The second greatest cause is tobacco, and alcohol is on the third place. Unhealthy food, tobacco, and alcohol are the three major causes of all health problems known to man, including obesity.

If you understand and accept this otherwise undeniable fact, then you have already found the solution to your problem. Yes, in order to lose weight, you need to deal with all the three main causes of illness, death and suffering of the modern society.

The two dominant causes of death, as far as diseases are concerned, are cardio-vascular diseases (heart diseases) and cancer. Both of these are caused primarily by unhealthy food, tobacco, and alcohol consumption, together with lack of physical activity, stress, and other causal factors. But again, the main cause is the food we eat. It is simple as that. And obese people are at much higher risk of almost all diseases, especially cardio-vascular diseases.

As far as these other causes of obesity are concerned, such as the mentioned endocrine system disorders, involving hypothalamus, pineal gland, or the pancreas, it really does not matter too much in treating obesity and losing weight, or any other health issue, because the underlying cause is all the same. The endocrine system disfunction was caused by wrong food intake over a long period of time. If you ingested toxins from other sources beside food, then the problem gets worsened.

It does not matter what organ will be hit mostly by the accumulated toxins coming from food and other sources, and it does not matter what hormonal changes and body responses will occur because of that. Moreover, it does not even matter what disease might appear, and how it is called among the medical doctors. None of it matters if you are aware that **the only or the main underlying cause of any sort of disharmony of your physical and/or mental health is the nutrient-deprived food you eat**.

Does genetics have something to do with obesity?

Many claimed that obesity was caused by a genetic disorder, that it had genetic origin. What they were trying to say was that you couldn't do anything about it. It's simply you, and you cannot change that condition – so they said.

Nothing could be further from the truth. Obesity is NOT caused by any genetic disorder, at least not in case of majority of obese people. And even if it was caused by some genetic disorder, it would still not mean you couldn't lose weight. You can and you will.

The question of relation between genes and obesity is actually completely irrelevant. Do not even bother thinking abou it. It does not matter whether you have obese parents, or if all your family members are obese. The potential connection between genes and obesity, or any disease and health problem in general, is irrelevant. It is irrelevant for two reasons: First, ALL health problems have partly a genetic origin, that is, certain genes are responsible for certain body functions that are damaged due to certain diseases; but this does not mean those diseases are inherited through genes, or that they cannot be cured, that it's all predetermined and that you just can't do anything about it. And secondly, genes certainly have something to do with you being obese, but again, it does not mean your obesity was primarily caused by some either normal or abnormal genes. It only means that you have a certain degree of genetic predisposition for becoming obese, and despite that predisposition, you can still lose weight and become slim.

Closest to the truth would be the statement that our **body shape** is of pure genetic origin, just like our height, skull shape, length of legs, the color of our eyes and hair, etc. Simply, some of us have a large neck and shoulders, a robust body, while others are naturally thin and of smaller stature. That is quite normal and has nothing to do with someone being obese and his ability to lose weight. All it means, this whole story about genes, is that we differ in body shape, and nothing more than that.

In cases of claimed genetic origin of certain health problems, the truth of the matter is that there is again only a genetic predisposition for the health problems in question, which does not necessarily mean those health problems will ever appear. And they won't; they will never show up IF we don't let it happen by our own choices we make concerning the food we eat, the water and other beverage we drink, and everything else we ingest, and all we do in our life. A famous American doctor once said that all health problems were caused by a mixture of our genetics and our lifestyle, in 50:50 proportion, adding that the health problem will never show up just because of genetics, that is, because our genetic predisposition to some health problem, be it obesity or anything else. The genetic predisposition will only become "activated" if we enable its activation by our diet and lifestyle.

This means that even if have no genetic predisposition to obesity or any other health problem, but we live an unhealthy life, we will still be in danger of becoming obesity or falling ill. The point is that it all depends on our behavior. The argument about the alleged genetic origin of obesity is only an excuse of nutritionists and doctors who failed to teach others how to lose weight and become healthy.

There is also one more thing caused partially by genes; it is your **body metabolism**. This mainly refers to time needed for food to be processed in your stomach and absorbed in your bowels. If the metabolism is slow, then you gain weight faster than others, even if you do not eat too much; and if it is faster, you don't gain weight even if you eat a lot and too often.

Since it is partially determined by genes, does it mean that the level of your body metabolism has nothing to do with you and your choices? No, since genes play only a minor role. If you are obese, you definitely have a slow, **low metabolism**, without any question, which means that you gain weight much faster and more easily than other people do, even if you don't eat too much and too often.

Again, however, this does not mean you can't do anything about it, that you can't change it. It does not matter if your low metabolism or anything else concerning your body and your health is genetically determined or not, because none of those things can stop you from losing weight; it can all be improved and solved. Your low metabolism only means that your body does not process food and absorb its ingredients fast enough, but it can be changed anyway, and must be changed in order to lose weight.

You can guess what the main cause of low metabolism actually is – Yes, it is again the nutrient-deprived food we eat every day. Of course, there are many other causes, but they are all related to eating and other daily habits, which we will discuss in this book. All in all, **genetics does not play any important role in obesity problem** you should consider and think about. All you will need to do is to address the problem of your food, and think about what you eat, what you drink, what you inhale, and what you do in everyday life, because those are the things that cause obesity and other health problems, not genetics.

Fake or inefficient weight-loss diets as one of the main causes of obesity

You have probably heard about myriad of different diets. A friend told you about a diet; a nutritionist or a doctor suggested another diet; your read about some new diet in newspapers, heard it on TV, or saw it on the Internet, perhaps you read some books about different diets, and so on. Many of those diets have something in common, while there are many completely different diets, and among them some quite unusual ones.

Some of them emphasize low-fat food, other diets emphasize low-carb food, then, some other diets promote the opposite – extremely high-fat or high-carb food, vegetarian-based, fruit-based, and countless other diets. How can you know which one is the true diet that will help you lose weight? Why are there so many diets anyway? Is it an individual matter – one diet is good for you, but other diets are good for someone else?

The answer to the last question must be "No". It is not an individual matter; if the cause of obesity is one and the same, as it is, then the solution must be one and the same for everyone, that is, the weight-loss diet must be one and the same for all obese people. Then why are there so many different weight-loss diets, and when I say different, I really mean an enormous number of completely different diets?

Well, let's put it this way: If you asked a historian to tell you about the beginnings of history, when did it all begin, when did the first human beings came to be, you will get a great number of completely different answers, ranging from a couple of thousand of years to a couple of millions of years. Some historians will say it happened not more than 10.000 years ago, while others will claim it happened 500.000 years ago, and yet some of them will assert that they know the exact date. If you heard so many different answers, what would be your logical conclusion? How can you know which answer is true?

If ten historians give you ten different answers to your simple question about the beginning of history, it means **they do not know the answer**. In the same way, if ten nutritionists give you ten different diets to try, it means **they do not know what diet will help you lose weight**. Just think about it. Isn't that an obvious, logical, and only possible conclusion?

They are only testing different things that may or may not have helped some people at some point of time, and that one usually just temporarily. Therefore, the real question is, why would you listen to any of them? Why would you accept their claims and try something you are not 100% sure that it will work, something that you did not conclude and concurred with by your own common sense? Why would you try weight-loss diets that didn't make any breakthrough?

How do you know that? Well, if it did, and if it was true it would help you lose weight, then today there would be less overweight people, wouldn't it? Probably every single person in the world who has trouble with obesity would like to lose weight and try any diet if he knows it will help him doing it.

Today, there is more information about obesity, more knowledge about the anatomy of our body, and more weight-loss diets, than ever before in the whole humankind history. Considering this fact, there should be less obese and sick people than in times past; yet, the situation is quite the opposite: Today, there are more overweight people than ever before! What does that tell you?

Not only the number of overweight people, but also the number of really obese people has been increasing for decades. Today, there are more obese people than ever before. (The difference between overweight and obese is not that important, and we will hereafter consider them equal terms for the purpose of this book.)

Likewise, statistics tell us that there are more sick people today than ever before. There is a greater number of diseases than ever before. More and more people die every year because of various health problems, both the ones related to obesity and those that are not. How can anyone claim today, as they do claim, that medicine and science in general has progressed over the last few decades? If it was really true, then there would be less sick people, and yet we see that everything is quite the opposite.

Some people even think that opening new hospitals and pharmacies is a great thing, not realizing that the increasing number of both hospitals and pharmacies proves once more that there are more and more sick people, so much more that there isn't enough room for everyone in the existing hospitals!

Concerning some of the most famous and promoted diets, you certainly heard of the so-called low-fat diet. You might have tried it. They say, since you have an excess of fat in your body, then you should eat food which contains less fat, or almost no fat at all. However, the truth is that this concept does not make any sense. You need fat. Your body needs fat as energy reserves and for other purposes. Fats are necessary nutrients. Many people who tried low-fat diet did not succeed in losing weight, and those who did eat fat-rich diet did not necessarily gained more weight.

The same goes for the low-carb diet. They say, you need to eat less carbo-hydrates (sugars), "you must not eat bread", avoid cereals, and so on. However, the truth is that bread and grain in general should be the foundation of your diet. If you had to eat only one type of food for the rest of your life, in order to survive, you would have to choose bread. If you would pick any other food, you would very quickly get sick from nutrient deficiency and die after a very short time from hunger and diseases.

The Roman soldiers, who had to march for thousands of miles, usually had only raw wheat with them. That's what they mostly ate during the times of war, and only with this food they were able to conquer their enemies. Besides, if the low-carb diet is an ideal weight-loss diet, then what about those people who eat a lot of carbo-hydrates every day and yet they are thin?

The point is that none of the existing diets proved universally successful. Moreover, despite some of the benefits that some of them do give, many of those diets, especially the starving diets, actually only worsen the problem and make you more obese. How's that possible? When you are on a diet that starves you out, your body will start accumulating fat more than usual as a reserve during the time you feel a strong hunger because of the diet. In other words, your body will "think" you are in a life-threatining situation with little or no food left, so everything you eat then, no matter what kind of food and how small amounts of it, it will almost all automatically turn into fat.

Yes, you might lose a few pounds while you are on some of those diets, but some time after that, you will again gain more weight, even more than you had before the diet! So, dieting that way will actually make you more obese, because your body will turn "the survival mode" on, in order to keep everything functioning normally as it should and prepare itself for the survival situation your body "expects".

Any weight-loss diet you try will have the same effect as any food you ate until then – it will keep you hungry all the time and it will create the vicious circle from which you will hardly be able to escape. So, you will eat the prescribed (wrong) food, and you will feel hungry because of eating that food; then, you will want to eat more of that food, which will still not satisfy your hunger, and so on. It's almost the same thing as in case of eating the food you ate before and because of which you gained weight, the only difference being the type and amount of food you eat while on the diet.

It is obvious that in both cases you ate the wrong food lacking most or some of the nutrients your body needs. Basically, all popular diets are either inefficient or not weight-loss diets at all. And on top of everything, most of the diets worsen the problem, even when you lose weight while on the diet, because after that you again reach or outreach your previous body weight, resulting in more health problems and loss of will and motivation.

It is easy to lose weight, but can you keep it that way?

The essential problem of the popular weight-loss diets is that their promoters prescribe a diet that is intended only for losing weight while on the diet, meaning it is not something an average healthy person should and could eat for a longer period, or for any period. The moment you stop with the diet, you will re-gain the lost weight. This jo-jo effect has detrimental effect on both your physical and mental health, causing metabolism disorders, stomach and bowel problems, high blood pressure, high blood sugar level, and many potential diseases, on one side, and depression and emotional disorders, on the other side.

Again, the weight-loss diet is almost the same as the food you ate before, the food that made you obese; because in both cases it is almost the same as not eating any food at all. In both cases you feel hungry all the time, in both cases your body is starving, and in both cases you feel miserable, tired, and irritated.

Of course you will lose weight while on any of those weight-loss diets; your body is literally starving, you are not eating enough, and you are not eating the proper food you need. Of course anyone who does not eat food will lose weight, be it not eating the proper food or not eating at all. The only difference is that in the case of not eating anything, you will lose weight and fall ill faster.

Just like no sane man would completely abstain from eating food so that he could lose weight, in the same way nobody should be on those "weight-loss diets" just so that he could lose weight. With those diets you indeed can lose weight, but only temporarily and at the expense of your overall health.

It is a very easy task to lose weight, but the real question is, how to keep going that way, how to never gain weight again? It is true that you can lose weight rather quickly with just a little effort and self-control, by adhering to your weight-loss diet and with a few advices from a nutritionist and perhaps a psychologist, if you have emotional problems with being obese. However, none of it will ever solve the root cause of the problem, and in all these cases, you will very probably re-gain your old weight.

The point is not only in losing weight, which is easy (no matter if you don't believe it now); **the point is in losing weight without too much effort**, without feeling hungry all the time, and without being tired, nervous, agitated, moody, and depressed. The point is in losing weight once and for all and not re-gaining your old weight, which means **overcoming the abnormal desire for food**. Of course, not the desire for food itself, since we all must eat and since it is normal to feel hunger when not eating any food for a few hours, but overcoming the constant desire for low-nutrient food full of added toxins and the constant abnormal feeling of hunger. The constant hunger and constant eating even when you are not hungry are two things that make you obese.

That is why the point is to neutralize those two – constant hunger and eating when you are not hungry, a phenomenon usually styled "emotional eating", or emotional craving for food. It is a condition when you are trying to satisfy your needs with food only, as if you were inloved with food, so to say. Of course there is nothing wrong in enjoying a nice meal, but if you are trying to fulfill all your needs, including the inner need of feeling content, with your food, then you will have problems: All you will achieve is gain more weight, become more depressed, and you will never satisfy your hunger and that inner need, because **food serves only to fulfill your physiological need for food**, that is, hunger, not your psychological and emotional needs.

So, how to neutralize the emotional craving and constant hunger? Since the primary cause of that condition is the low-nutrient food you eat, then the solution is to start eating the food that contains all nutrients your body needs. If this sounds simple to you, know that it really is.

Likewise, it is important to know that there is another cause of eating when you are not hungry and feeling hunger at other times; it is a cause of emotional nature, or better to say, mental nature. We will talk a bit about mentality in a separate chapter of this book.

For now, the most relevant thing here for you to know is that your feeling of constant hunger, and your habit of eating too much, even when you don't feel hunger, CAN be neutralized, and you CAN lose weight without ever experiencing these two and all other symtpoms of impaired physical and emotional/mental health, such as depression, nervousness, agitation, tiredness, and so on. It is possible to do it without much effort, without feeling hungry all the time, without being tired all day long, and without extreme food restrictions. In one word: **You can be cured of the abnormal desire for food and lose all the weight you want!** Just keep reading and you will find out the answer. It's right here at the reach of your hand…

The problem of the food content

As already said, the food most people eat is the main problem; its content and the way it was produced. Its content is problematic because it does not contain nutrients your body needs, and on the other side, it does contain all possible non-nutrient substances that your body does not need at all, and moreover, those substances must not be present in your body under any circumstances.

Exactly those non-nutrient substances found in the food from stores are the main cause of obesity, beside other substances you ingest via water, sodas, juices, alcohol, air, or in any other way. What are those substances and why are they found in food we eat?

Those are artificially made substances for making the food taste good and stay longer on the shelves before spoiling. These substances are additives, conservants, flavor-enhancers, and many other chemical compounds that were not supposed to be in our food, and that should not be ingested, because **all those substances contain toxins, which cause obesity, food-addiction, and numerous health problems**.

If you think about it, you will realize that no normal healthy food in the world could stay on the shelves for too long. Any food will spoil in a very short time; but then how is it possible it didn't spoil? The answer is obvious: It didn't spoil because it did not contain almost any nutrient, because it was "empty food", and because it contained chemicals (read: toxins) that prolonged its expiration date. And those chemicals in that food are the ones that make you obese.

As for flavor-enhancers, it is a well-known fact how much those are detrimental to your health. All they do is make the food taste better and make you addicted to it. Yes, **the food sold today at stores contains chemicals that literally cause addiction**. That's another vicious circle created by the food you eat: You eat the food that contains food-addicting chemicals; you become hungry because of that food and crave for more; you eat that food, and then it makes you crave for more of that food, and so on. There is no end. It's like the story about a dragon that was becoming hungrier every time he ate something.

The thing about these substances is that they can make even the most gross food taste like your favorite food. If you injected those substances in trash, the trash would be tasteful! Actually, it's not really tasteful, it's just a taste you became addicted to because of the addiction-causing chemicals it contains. You can get used to any taste of almost any food.

The most (in)famous flavor-enhancer is **Monosodium-glutamate**, more commonly known as **MSG**. This substance is probably found in literally ALL food sold at stores. It enhances the flavor of all food, and perhaps is the primary or only reason why the nutrient-deprived food sold at stores has any taste at all! It is considered to be a type of the so-called excitotoxin – toxins that damage your brain cells and cause many health issues. There is a lot of data in scientific literature about excitotoxins, and many books have been written about MSG and similar toxins found in food.

Glutamate actually exists in our body, just like cholesterol. It is one of the brain chemicals. However, there is no need to take in glutamate from outside sources, especially not in the form of MSG-like substances – the same way there is no need to take in cholesterol from outside sources, especially not in the form of processed animal food containing additives, because the liver produces enough cholesterol our body needs.

Finally, besides many other toxic substances put into the food sold at stores, there is one special substance which make you obese: It is the **growth hormone**. The growth hormone gets injected into animals, so that the owners of animal farms could raise bigger animals and earn money faster and more easily. The meat and other products made from that animal are sold in stores, and people consume the products made from that animal, products that still retain the growth hormone injected into the body of the animal. And, you can guess, the growth hormone now affects your body in a similar way, making you more obese.

Together with growth hormone, they also give antibiotics to animals, and many other drugs, because those animals in large farms are all sick due to physical inactivity and food with which they are fed. Their food is actually similar to food we eat concerning its nutrient and toxic content. Did you know that **more than 50% of all produced antibiotic drugs is actually used for treating animals**?

Isn't it obvious that food products made from those animals should never be put for consummation? How can eating food made from sick animals full of growth hormone and toxins be good for people and not make them obese? How could possibly any food at stores which contains artificially made substances and toxins be good for people and not make them obese?

It's all plain and simple: The food you eat mainly consists of things that make you obese, and that's why you are obese. You might ask, then how come other people who eat the same food as you are not obese like you? This is where other causal factors come in, including the genes: You might have a certain level of genetic predisposition inherited from your parents for becoming obese quicker than other people, and more probably, you are less physically active than others, and you might do more of the other things that make you obese. We will mention them later in the book.

So, your diet mainly consists of harmful substances, artificial taste-enhancers, and other toxic chemicals they inject in food and that make you obese and cause numerous health issue; or better to say what your food does NOT contain and it should – The food you eat does not contain nutrients and any thing that your body needs. It contains everything else your body does not need, everything that harms your body, creating a metabolism disorder which causes obesity.

The problem of the food industry

The harmful toxic effects of MSG, growth hormone, additives, taste-enhancers, and all other chemicals they put in the food we eat, are well-known and fully researched. There is no question about it. You do not have to be an expert in anything to realize that the food we eat is literally poisoned by insecticides and every other toxic substance used by food producers, and by toxic substances added by food product manufacturers. Likewise, you do not have to be an expert to know that the refined processed food we buy every day is unhealthy and genetically modified, that it lacks all nutrients, that it contains many harmful chemicals, that it causes many health problems, and that **it is the main cause of obesity**.

A common sense is enough to tell you that it really is so. You do not need "an expert" to tell you what the truth is. You do not need anyone to explain you the food content, and you do not need anyone to convince you that the food is not the main cause of obesity, and that there is some other way of losing weight beside not eating that kind of food, but that there is some shortcut to losing weight, some "magical formula" or "a magical pill". **The only way to lose weight is to stop**

eating the nutrient-deprived MSG-added GMO toxic food sold at stores.

Before we move onto the topic about the food you should eat in order to lose weight, there is one question left to be answered: Why do they put the chemicals into our food that make you obese, even though they know those chemicals cause obesity and other health problems? Of course, the answer to this question does not matter too much, since it doesn't change a thing about the content of the food which makes you obese; nevertheless, the answer is rather obvious. They put those chemicals in our food for several reasons:

First, they need to put the chemicals in so that the food could stay on the shelves for a longer period; otherwise, it would quickly become spoiled. Secondly, they need to put the taste-enhancers in so that the food could have any taste, and so that they could force the consumers to buy that food. Also, they put chemicals in food because those chemicals cause addiction to food; that way, too, they force you to buy and eat the food they produce. And finally, many food producers have contracts signed with pharmaceutical companies, so when they put chemicals in the food that causes obesity and other health problems, you afe forced to buy medications for those health problems which are produced by the said pharmaceuticals companies. There is nothing strange and secret about it. As a matter of fact, it is a so well-known information that they mention it even in the schoolbooks.

Anyone could see that the main reason for putting harmful chemicals in food by food producers is the profit. By using these tricks of chemistry and propaganda through commercials, the food producers sell more and more of their unhealthy food, causing obesity and other health problems, which in turn make people buy medications produced by pharmaceutical companies that are allied with the same food producers. For example, a producer of chocolate might have a contract with a producer of toothpaste or antihistamines (anti-allergic) medications, because chocolate causes tooth decay and allergies, especially among children; that way, they gain even more profit through their mutual cooperation, at the expense of our health.

I believe there is much more involved in that inhuman business than money, but let's not get into the story and touch the subject of the so-called conspiracy theories. The point is that the food they willingly produce that way is unhealthy, that it causes obesity and diseases, and that the only possible way to get healthy and lose weight is to stop eating the food they produce. There is simply no other way to do it.

The problem of the drugs industry

The problem is not only in the cooperation between food companies which produce unhealthy food and the pharmaceutical industry producing medications which treat the health problems caused by that food; but the main problem is that **the medications they produce for treating those health problems, actually, cause more health problems** because of their content and side-effects.

In this way, there is yet another vicious circle going on: You eat the unhealthy food which causes obesity and other health problems; because of that, you take medications, which cause other health problems; then, you take other medications for treating those other health problems, and at the same time you eat more of the food that causes health problems, and so on.

It is a well-known and undeniable fact that ALL medications have side-effects, treating one organ, while causing damage to other organs, especially the liver and colon. There is always a long list of their side-effects, and their content of numerous chemicals is enough to prove their toxicity. Therefore, if you are taking any medication at this moment, you are also ingesting many harmful substances found in it, despite the medication's possible temporal beneficial effects. By taking medications you are actually causing more damage to your health, and you acidify (toxify) your blood and clog your organs, making it less possible to lose weight. In other words, **medications delay the positive outcome and make losing weight a more difficult task, while some of them even contribute to gaining more weight**.

The other problem of pharmaceutical drugs is that **they only treat the symptoms of the health problem in question, but they do not treat its cause**, meaning they are not even designed for the purpose of curing diseases. For example, if you have a headache, a doctor will give you a drug that alleviates the pain, but will never treat the very cause of headache; and the cause of headache might be coffee and cigarettes. In this case, the real cure for the headache, that is, a health problem with a headache as a symptom, could only be quitting coffee and cigarettes. So, there is practically no reason to take medications for every possible health problem, since they will cause damage more than they will cure you of any health problem, besides making it harder for you to lose weight.

It is a better solution to use natural methods of healing which have no side-effect and do not involve taking any chemical and artificially made substances. Moreover, if you stick to the weight-loss program described in the next chapter, you will never need any medication, because you will lose all the weight you want and be completely healthy.

Now, the question is, are you ready to do it? Are you ready to make some changes in your diet and lifestyle, and in all your daily habits? Are you really ready to lose weight once and for all, knowing that you do not need to struggle with your hunger and put too much effort in it, and knowing that you will surely lose weight in a very short period? All you will have to do is just stop eating the poisoned food and make a few simple changes in your life, so simple, that you will greatly wonder why you have not done it before, and how come you never heard about it before.

Let's get it started!

THE WEIGHT-LOSS PROGRAM

What are those changes you have to make? As I said, just some simple changes, something you might call trivial, but it's actually essential for losing weight, becoming 100% healthy, and full of energy and life spirit. It's something that actually makes you alive, in the full sense of that word, that will revive your spirit and your physical condition, something what our body is designed for, something that you are designed for…

This weight-loss program involves only 7 simple changes in your life. That is why there are 7 separate book chapters discussing each of the steps. These are the seven changes you should make:

1) The first thing is **WATER**. Why is water in the first place? Shouldn'the food be in the first place? The water holds the first spot because it is the most essential physiological need, a life need, without which we can hardly survive for two days.
   Believe it or not, plain natural water is the essence and the key to losing weight. No tricks about it, no special usage of water, nothing special and mysterious about it, just some plain water you drink every day is needed for losing weight.
   Hey, if someone told you that you would lose weight or solve some health problem only by drinking water, would you heed this advice, would you not try it? Wouldn't it be the first thing you would do, since it sounds way too simple and requires no effort at all? I assure you that you will start losing weight the moment you hear the story about the water below.

2) The second change concerns **SUN and AIR** – another two elements of nature. And all you have to do is expose your body to sunlight and fresh clean air, and you need only to change one thing about **BREATHING**.
   How hard can it be? This sounds even simpler than all the rest, doesn't it? Yet, there is nothing special about it: No tricks and some special "breathing exercises", sungazing, and meditation; just some plain breathing you will hear about in a separate

chapter of this book. And again, believe it or not, this WILL help you lose weight.

3) The third change concerns **PHYSICAL ACTIVITY**. Let me say it right at the start: Without enough physical activity, you simply CANNOT lose weight. Physical activity is as essential as water and food both for losing weight and staying healthy. But do not worry at the slightest; you will not have to run, jump, and do exercices all day long seven times a week. For the start, just a bit of plain and simple walking will do the job. Can you believe it?

4) The fourth change is all about **REST**. Rest? Should not someone who is obese be more physically active? Certainly, but still this not does not mean you will be active throughout the whole day and even practice and go jogging at night. You need to rest, too, and rest in a proper way. We are talking about a classic rest in bed, nothing more. It cannot get any simpler than that.

5) The fifth change is all about **MENTALITY** and spirituality. In treating any physical condition, including obesity, mental health must be in check, too. It is equally important to be mentally and spiritually healthy as it is to be physically healthy and in good condition.
What does this imply? Again, nothing exceptional you should worry about. All it means is that you should treat the causes of your stress, if any, and that you should read some quality books or watch inspirational videos, listen to appropriate music, hang out with good positive-thinking people, and so on. Read, watch, and talk about good things – I don't think you will believe this in the beginning, before you see the results.

6) The sixth change concerns the **FOOD**, that is, your diet. We would all agree this is the most important part of the program, though the previous five are perhaps equally important. The diet is "the first among equals", as they say.

What food you should eat? Again, nothing exceptional about it. There are no tricks, no shortcuts, no "special diets", no starving, no feeling hungry all the time, no jo-jo effect, no nothing. Just some plain simple food you should eat. And you can eat bread, and fruit, and vegetable, and beans, and nuts, and meat, and dairy, and anything else, as much as you want. Alright, I am not saying you should eat literally everything, since we are not omnivores; for example, you should not eat the MSG food sold at stores, which I described on the previous pages, but almost all other things are available to you.

7) And last, but not least, is **BOWEL CLEANSE**. This one should actually be done before anything else, but I put it in the last place because the first six in this list are the simplest steps, while this one includes a few things to remember that you have probably never done in your life. It's not complicated, either, it's just a simple method of cleansing the constipated bowels. Though I said "bowel cleanse", it actually involves the cleansing of other organs, too, such as the liver. Bowel cleanse is the most important one. It is the foundation of this program. However, other organs should be cleansed, as well. That way, you will lose weight much more easily and quickly.

If you follow these steps and this simple weight-loss program, which does not require any particular effort and self-sacrifice, you will most definitely lose weight in a very short period. There is 0% chance you will not succeed IF you stick to the program. Even if you don't do it all as you should, even if you sometimes ignore some of the steps, you will still lose weight to some extent. However, I advise you to do it all the way through; because it is easy and it will help you get your desired weight.

Follow me through these pages; you are only steps away from getting your desired weight in the easiest way possible. You are exactly seven steps away!

1. WATER

The first step of the weight-loss program is water. What about it? There are a few quite simple things to know and remember about water regarding obesity.

The most important thing to know is that up to 75% of our body is made of water. This statement is not important for you just so that you could know why we can't live without water for too long, but it's important because it tells us that **we must drink a lot of water every day**.

We all know that, someone might say; but do we?

Actually, the truth is that **the majority of people do not drink enough water**. It may be true in your case, too. An American doctor said that **if people drank more water every day, there would be much less obese people, and about 80% of diseases would not exist**! Can you believe this statement? Just a few more cups of water every day, and there would be so much less of health problems and suffering.

If we don't drink enough water, dehydration ensues, causing immunity decline, which in turn causes you to get sick more quickly. Without enough water in your body, your blood flow becomes slower, your bowels become clogged, your liver becomes clogged, and all your other organs become clogged, and the whole body starts choking in the accumulated toxins that have not been flushed out by water.

An acidic toxic body environment causes and worsens obesity, not letting you lose weight permanently and get rid of the abnormal desire for food. That is why you must start drinking more water every day. From now on you should **drink at least 6-8 glasses of plain clean water each day** on a normal wheather day and when not too physically active. And during the hot summer days, or when more physically active, you should drink more than that. If you drink enough water during the day, your urine should be colorless; and if it has yellow color, strong smell, or foamy consistence, you should drink more water. (Foamy consistence indicates an excess of animal protein intake.)

Each morning when you wake up, the first thing to do is to drink a glass of water. That should be the first thing to do the moment you wake up, and it should become your daily habit from now on. Just by doing this – drinking 6-8 glasses of water every day – you will initiate the process of losing weight. Can you believe it? Indeed, it is true, and it cannot get any simpler than that.

However, there is this other thing to remember: **You should never drink tap water**, for the reason of its content. Without question and a shroud of doubt, the tap water is full of harmful chemicals and toxins, just like the food sold at stores. Do not drink tap water, only take bottled water or use well and natural sources of clean water, if those are available to you. If not, then drink bottled water. However, you should beware of bottled water, as well, since they add fluoride and chlorine, so the safest way is to use water filters, such as RO water filter or reversible osmosis filter. You can even drink distilled water, no matter it is deprived of some of the minerals regular water contains.

Also, it is very important to remember when NOT to drink water:

- You should never drink water with your meal.
- You should never drink water just before the meal.
- You should never drink water just after the meal.

You can drink water only **an hour after the last meal** you had. The same applies to any other liquid, such as juices or teas. If you drink something during the meal, right before it, or during the first hour after the meal, you will dilute the stomach acid and disrupt the food digestion process, slowing it down and increasing the chance of your food getting stuck in the bowels to spoil and release toxins directly into your blood. The whole water scenario worsens the problem of obesity.

A hydrotherapy method

And finally, water can be applied externally. Besides regular bathing, there is a special use of water – hydrotherapy, which might be of help in losing weight.

The standard external use of water for increasing blood circulation is the **application of hot and cold water**. You, too, can apply this simple natural hydrotherapy method. By increasing blood circulation all through your body and speeding up your metabolism rate, this method will help you in losing weight more quickly and feeling more energetic.

All you have to do is to apply hot shower for 1 minute and cold shower for 30 seconds; then, 1 minute of hot shower and 30 seconds of cold shower again; and do it this way a couple of times, not more than seven times. You can apply the shower all over your body.

Of course, you should not use too hot water, so hot to burn your skin; and you should not use ice cold water. Just apply the hottest and coldest water possible, the hottest and coldest you can endure, but do not overdo it. Use your sense of reason and start first with the milder temperature difference. Do not apply it to your head, and first start with the legs, slowly and gradually increasing or decreasing the water temperature, until your body adapts to it.

Who would say that a simple application of hot and cold water will help in losing weight? Who would ever think that plain consummation of water "burns" the fat in your stomach?

2. SUN AND AIR

The second step of the weight-loss program – sun and air. Basically, all you have to do is to **expose your skin to sunlight more often and spend more time on clean fresh air**. It does sound too simple, but there are a few ideas you should take into consideration...

Regarding the exposure to sunlight, you should do it at least 15 minutes a day. It is the minimum. However, an hour of "sunbath" a day is a better choice; and it would be far better if you do it for more than an hour, and spend time outdoors as much as possible. Beside many beneficial effects of the sunlight, such as prevention of depression and bone diseases (osteoporosis), it is a well-known fact that skin exposed to sunlight produces vitamin D, so that you do not need any food source or a vitamin supplement.

If you spend too much time indoors, it's time to change that habit and expose your skin to sunlight more often. As you'll see in the next chapter, in order to lose weight, you will have to be more physically active, so you will have to spend more time outdoors anyway.

The same goes for breathing in clean fresh air. In order to do that, you just need to spend more time outdoors. It would be even better if you could spend more time in the countryside, especially in a mountain area, where the air is clean and fresh, in any case, better than the air in city areas.

I knew a young man who was cured only by breathing in fresh air: He was feeling sick and weak all the time, but when he went to visit some cousins who lived on a high mountain, he had a strange experience; he suddenly started feeling more energetic, but was constantly coughing and had an unbelievable nose-running. Huge amounts of liquid were coming out from his nose non-stop. What happened, you wonder? It was the clean fresh mountain air that initiated the process of body cleansing and self-healing process. Next day the nose-running stopped and he felt amazing. Therefore, do not underestimate the significance of the fresh air.

But what does it have to do with someone being overweight? Well, besides it is beneficial for your overall health, you should be aware that the oxygen burns fat; more oxygen you inhale, more fat is burned, so that you lose more weight.

You could also do some breathing exercises, although I would not recommend some "special" exercises, involving meditation, background music, falling into some kind of trance, or anything of the kind. Just a bit of plain and simple deep breathing. That's all.

3. PHYSICAL ACTIVITY

Related to sun and air exposure, physical activity makes the third step of the weight-loss program. As already said, without it, you CANNOT lose weight. Actually, without physical activity, you cannot even be healthy. Our body is designed to be physically active all the time.

Physical activity can include walking, fast-walking, jogging, swimming, playing football or some other sport, working in the garden, in the field, in the woods, at work, at home, and so on. The best and most suitable activity for overweight and obese people is **walking**.

So, all you would have to do is to **start walking for at least an hour every day**. It does not have to be fast, there is nothing special about it, just some plain walking for an hour, either alone or with someone. No need for hard exercises, exhausting yourselves, or jumping and running all day long. Walk, walk, and walk, every day for an hour. Even if you do not have to go anywhere, you should walk toward any place you want and then come back the same way.

I would also recommend **working in the garden**, if you have one, since it is one of the best and healthiest physical activities. All muscles in the body are active during the gardening, and you can take short breaks whenever you want. Also, by having a garden of your own, you can produce food for yourself, and in that way avoid buying the unhealthy food at stores that make you obese.

Physical activity increases blood circulation and metabolism rate, as well as oxygen intake, which helps in losing weight. Also, physical activity is necessary for maintaining your well-being and mental health, and represents the best natural cure for depression. Therefore, be more physically active and spend time outdoors exposed to sun and fresh air, in order to get your desired weight.

It is recommended to be physically active during the day, not at sunset or at night, since your body needs to prepare for the night rest and sleeping at that time. If you are physically active at night, then your body will not be able to rest properly, and then your metabolism rate will decrease, making it harder to lose weight, and your immunity response will become weak, making you more prone to diseases. That is why it is important to be physically active during the day while the sun is still there shining upon you, and at night to have a proper rest...

4. REST

After physical activities during the day on fresh air, your body and mind need to rest. No matter if it sounds untrue or contradictory to you, but a rest in bed can help you lose weight. How so?

It's not just any kind of rest. Of course that you will gain weight if you rest all day and do nothing. I am talking about resting after physical activity, and I am talking about the proper rest. Improper and irregular rest leads to obesity and many other health problems, while the proper regular rest keeps you healthy and full of energy.

Resting helps you lose weight as a part of the whole weight-loss program, because if all parts of the program are implemented, then your body will start getting back into balance and revive its normal metabolism, initiating the processes that regulate your body weight. Simply put, if someone is too slim, he will start gaining weight a bit, and if someone is overweight, he will start losing weight. That's how it works.

What does a proper rest imply? It implies **going to bed at the right time, 10-11 PM at the latest**, and getting up at the right time, that is, **sleeping for 6-8 hours**. It is true someone needs to sleep more time than the others, while some people sleep little. However, it is important to go to bed before 11 PM because you need to reach the so-called REM sleep phase (the deepest sleep) before 2 AM. Why?

It's because of one hormone that is being produced in your brain during the night, called **melatonin**. It is a hormone which helps in regeneration and rejuvenation of your body. If you fail to go to bed on time, you will disrupt its production in the brain, and that way you will not be able to get a proper rest, but you will wake up all tired and moody. If you wake up feeling tired, it means you disrupted the sleep cycle by improper rest, although it could also and more probably indicate unhealthy diet. The same goes for sleeping during the day; you should avoid it.

A proper rest at night also implies sleeping in a completely quiet room, without a TV on, without listening to music before you fall asleep, without any light in the room (a complete darkness is necessary), and with good ventilation. A proper rest and physical activity alone will help you lose some weight, let alone if you implement the other five steps of this weight-loss program.

5. MENTALITY

The fifth step is mentality and spirituality – perhaps, it is the most important step of the program. Namely, it is impossible to stay physically healthy if your mental and spiritual health is not in check. For example, if you are feeling depressed most of the time, it means you have to work on your mentality and spirituality. I am not talking about any special "spiritual technique", or anything like it; just a few reasonable advices that concern your way of thinking and emotional state.

Knowing that this weight-loss program will help you lose weight, knowing that it cannot be any other way if you stick to it, there is no reason to be depressed, if you feel that way, because of your current weight and overall condition. There is no reason to lose hope and to think that you will never lose weight, no matter how much you were trying to lose weight before and how successful you were. Now you have more information and a new guide and set of rules to follow, which will most definitely make you lose weight almost without any effort. So, the first thing to remember is this: **Do not worry at all about your current weight**; it will change very soon.

The second equally important thing to remember concerns your way of thinking. You must think only about good, positive things; you should watch only good program, inspirational videos and movies; you should listen to good music with a positive message in the text of the song (no violent rhythm, loud music, vulgarity in the song…); you should read inspirational and motivational books with a positive message; you should hang out with good positive-thinking people and family members; and in short, you should do only good things that promote positive thinking and helping others in need.

You should never do these things: Have negative and pessimistic thoughts, watch violent and horror movies, listen to loud aggressive music, read occult or adult literature, and hang out with people who gossip and always criticize something or someone; because if you do any of these things, you will be unhappy and depressed, which will only worsen the problem of obesity and add to your emotional craving for food.

I would neither recommend reading romances nor anything else that will make you feel depressed or overflown with emotions; self-help books; and "mind map" books or anything related to psychology and similar subjects. Stay away from all those books, no matter where you heard about them or if your dear friend told you to read them.

Also, I would not recommend doing any kind of spiritual or relaxation techniques, yoga, meditation, and many other popular techniques used for "relaxing" and "stabilizing your mind", because all of those are simply psychological tricks for your mind, a kind of spiritual drugs that sedate your mind and spirit, but when their effect is over, you will feel again the same way as before, because those techniques cannot solve the root of any problem, but only treat the symptoms and give a temporal, very short (false) relief from stress – just like pharmaceutical drugs that only relieve symptoms of the disease, not the cause, and the exact same way the popular "weight-loss diets" only offer temporal loss of weight, plus a bunch of troubles in struggling with your hunger and emotional stress.

It is extremely important to avoid practicing of the above-mentioned techniques; but if you are much involved in spiritual and religious matters, then all you should do is simple **praying in your own words**. Perhaps, you could pray for strength to endure and succeed in losing weight and staying healthy, or overcoming the abnormal desire for food.

Overcoming the abnormal craving for food

I mentioned the abnormal desire for food and "emotional eating" in an earlier chapter in relation to nutrient-deprived food, saying that this kind of food and the fake weight-loss diets keep you hungry all the time and cause an emotional craving for food. However, the root cause of that craving is not the food itself, but your mental and emotional state, which means that the problem can only be solved in the above-explained manner, since you do not possess real strength in you to overcome something that is almost instinctive in your nature. To overcome the desire itself, you must get help from the outside source.

A wise man once asked: "Can a leopard change his spots? Or can people who are taught wrong do good?" And in the same way I ask: "Can people who crave for food all the time overcome their craving?" The answer is "No", not by their will alone, because it will require self-discipline and constant struggling with your thoughts and desires, just like when you are on a fake weight-loss diet. That way, you will not overcome the desire permanently. In truth, how could anyone overcome their own desires, how to defeat your own nature? Perhaps you could ponder more about spiritual matters…

Even if you are not religious at all, faith still matters, because **what you think about is what you get, and what you believe is how you behave**. Your faith determines your behavior. If you want to lose weight, you have to believe it is possible to do it, you must have faith in success. Studies have shown that religious people who had faith and strongly believed they would get cured of their health problems, really got cured faster than others and did not even went through much pain and struggle. The same is true in losing weight, though of course, you should follow all other steps of the program. And the last two steps will surely help in overcoming emotional craving for food and finally getting your desired weight.

6. FOOD

Understandably, the essential component of the weight-loss program is diet. Although there are no strict restrictions as in case of other weight-loss programs, still there is some food you should eat more, some food you should eat less, and some food you should avoid at all costs. The main problem with the diet of the majority of people is that they did the opposite and chose the wrong food to eat in plenty and wrong food to eat in smaller amounts. You probably did it, too, so all you have to do is to just make a few changes in your diet and eating habits.

Before speaking of what food to eat or not to eat, there are some rules about the right time for eating:

- **Always have a breakfast**. Overweight people, and other people in general, as by rule, rarely eat anything in the morning. Skipping a breakfast worsens the obesity problem and your health in general. A breakfast is the most important meal, so important that not only you must never skip it, but you should have a big meal for your breakfast.

- **Skip your dinner**. Dinner meal is not necessary. It is best to avoid it or eat only a small meal, some fruit, for example. Though many people are used to skipping a breakfast and having a big meal for a dinner, you must do the opposite from now on, in order to lose weight. It is not hard to do it, because if you start eating a big meal for every breakfast, you will feel no need for a large meal at night. If you only do this, if you always eat breakfast and skip your dinner meal, you will already start losing weight.

- **Your last meal must be at least 3.5 hours before going to bed**. The main reason for skipping dinner is the impossibility of digestion during the sleep. If you eat at night, and especially if you eat a large meal, the food will not be completely digested in your stomach, because the digestion process and your metabolism rate slows down at night and during the sleep. That way, partly digested food will remain in your bowels and clog the colon, making you constipated, which in turn causes obesity and many other health problems, including depression, as far as emotional health is concerned.

- **Eat 2-3 times a day**. Since you should have a large breakfast and avoid dinner, you should have 2 meals a day. Many dietitians and nutritionists would recommend either eating 3 times a day, or eating smaller meals at least 6 times a day. This is a completely wrong scenario, because that way your stomach muscle will never have a chance to rest, and all muscles in your body must rest. Therefore, you should eat only 2-3 times a day, and if you are very obese, it should be 2 times a day (without a dinner). Do not worry, you will not feel the abnormal hunger all the time, if you eat the right food I will discuss below. However, know that feeling a bit of hunger between meals is quite normal.

- **Make a pause of at least 5 hours between two meals**. This is necessary for your stomach muscle to digest all the food from the previous meal and to have time for rest. It would be best to eat a large breakfast meal early in the morning and a medium lunch meal 5-6 hours later, while skipping the dinner or eating only a light meal, such as fruit, at least 3.5-4 hours before going to bed. That way, you will be very hungry in the morning, when a large breakfast should await you.

A few more tips on eating habits:

- **Do not eat anything between meals**. Do not eat a snack or anything between the two main meals – a breakfast and a lunch, because that would prolong the digestion of food and make your stomach work without resting. Endure the temporal hunger in the beginning, so that your stomach could get used to the new (normal) regime. Besides, when you stop eating the processed food from stores, and instead start eating the right nutrient-rich food, you will feel no need for a snack between meals.

Your only "snack" between meals should be **water**. It would be great if you start carrying a small bottle of water wherever you go. Even if you are at home, you should always have that bottle of water in front of you. Let the water be your "temptation substitute" instead of food.

- **Eat slowly**. You should eat your food slowly and chew it well. This is very important to remember. Eating slowly will satisfy your hunger more quickly and will keep your stomach satisfied for a longer time.

- **Never mix fruit and vegetable in a single meal**, because it will cause stomach problems, flatulence, and diarrhea.

What food to avoid

Basically, it's almost all food sold at stores that you should avoid. As already explained in the first chapter, that kind of food contains many chemicals, toxins, and artificially-made substances that make you obese, cause addiction, and have very harmful effects on your overall health. Simply, the undeniable fact is that almost **all food sold at stores and super-markets is unhealthy food, unhealthy without exception, that is the main reason for you being obese and the main cause of disease and death**.

The only possible and the only true way of losing weight necessitates avoiding this food at all costs. You would need to stop buying it if you want to lose weight and be healthy. Instead, start buying the groceries in health-good stores, or a marketplace, from people you know to sell organically grown and chemical-free food, or better yet – make your own garden and start your own food production, if possible. At least try to do something about it, because simply there is no other way, there is no shortcut or a trick. You have to make some radical changes and decisions concerning your diet and other daily habits.

What food to eat

The only food you should not eat is the food sold at stores. All other food you are allowed to eat. Actually, you can eat the same food which is sold at stores, but not that exact food standing on the shelves in those stores. For example, you should not buy the white bread in a supermarket, but you can still eat bread; either buy the wholegrain bread, or make the wholegrain bread by yourself. Or if you want a juice, you can drink it, but do not buy the one from stores; just juice some organic fruit in a juicer.

You may eat almost any food and still lose weight: You may eat all fruit and vegetable, all grains (bread), all nuts, all legumes, all dairy products, and almost all meat. However, there is one rule on the percentage of each of these in your meals: Bread should be the foundation of every meal, and with it you can either eat fruit and nuts, or vegetable, nuts, legumes, dairy, and meat. In other words, either use fruit or vegetable with other ingredients, but never mix fruit and vegetable in the same meal. This is the list of appropriate meal combinations:

1) - Wholegrain cereals / bread (wheat, oat, buckwheat…);
   - Fruit (apple / banana / pear / orange…);
   - Nuts (hazelnuts / walnuts / Brazil nuts / peanuts…).

2) - Wholegrain cereals / bread (wheat, oat, buckwheat…);
   - Vegetable (tomato / carrot / cucumber…);
   - Nuts (hazelnuts / walnuts / Brazil nuts / peanuts…).

3) - Wholegrain cereals / bread (wheat, oat, buckwheat…);
   - Legumes (bean / pea / lentils…);
   - Vegetable (tomato / carrot / cucumber…).

4) - Wholegrain cereals / bread (wheat, oat, buckwheat…);
   - Fruit (apple / banana / pear / orange…);
   - Seeds (sunflower / pumpkin / sesame / soy…).

5) - Wholegrain cereals / bread (wheat, oat, buckwheat…);
   - Dairy product (yoghurt, milk, cheese…);
   - Vegetable (tomato / carrot / cucumber…).
   - Seeds (sunflower / pumpkin / sesame / soy…).

6) Wholegrain cereals / bread (wheat, oat, buckwheat…);
   - Vegetable (tomato / carrot / cucumber…).
   - Meat (chicken / fish / lamb…).

As you can see from the list, you can eat almost any food: Cereals or bread and fruit or vegetable with some nuts or seeds being your main food, with dairy products or meat sometimes altering the fruit.

However, it is important to know that you should not eat this food in great amounts: meat, meat products, milk and dairy products, and all food of animal origin, but the other vegetable food listed above must comprise the greatest percentage of your diet. Why so? There are at least three good reasons:

- First, that kind of food is rich in all nutrients your body needs;
- Secondly, that kind of food helps in losing weight faster;
- And thirdly, our body is designed for that kind of food, that is, our stomach and all other organs are designed for digesting that kind of food.

On relation between human anatomy and diet

Our body is designed for digesting vegetable food in the first place, since **human beings are herbivores according to their anatomy and physiology**. You might not like that, but it's simply a scientific fact, as I will show you.

For example, if you take a look at our teeth, you will plainly see that they look like the teeth of any herbivore animal – they are designed for grinding plant food. We do not have sharp teeth for tearing hard-digesting food like carnivores do. Also, our saliva is of the same chemical content as the saliva of other herbivores.

Our stomach acid is very mild, just like the stomach acid of herbivore animals, while carnivore animals have a very strong stomach acid. Next, our bowels are very long and "wrinkled", so to say, just like in case of all other herbivores, while carnivores possess short smooth bowels; that way, the hard-digesting food they eat could go through the bowels more quickly, so as not to cause the clogging of the bowels and poisoning.

Even if you take a look at our hands, you will see they are obviously designed for grabbing fruit, not for tearing some animal apart and eating its flesh. Certainly, we are adapted to eating animal food, too, but if we eat more animal than vegetable food, we gain weight and get sick. Though I am neither a vegetarian, nor am I telling you to become one, it is indeed a fact that a vegetarian or vegan diet is the fastest way of losing weight. Therefore, you should eat more vegetable than animal food.

This is not a starving diet, you will not be hungry all the time and your body will not lack any vitamin or other nutrient if you eat more vegetable food, as some people claim. No, you will get all the needed nutrients and you won't feel hungry all the time, like you do feel when you eat nutrient-deprived food or if you are on a "weight-loss diet". You won't feel hungry because you will eat very nutritious **wholegrain bread**, which will make you full really quickly, as well as other whole foods rich in all nutrients your body needs.

You can only feel abnormal and constant hunger if you do not supply your body with all the necessary nutrients, which are not present in the processed refined MSG food sold in bags and packages at stores. You will stay hungry only if you eat bread made of refined white flour, because only 7% of that bread contains important nutrients. **Lack of nutrients in the food you eat is the main reason why you can eat a lot and still not satisfy your hunger**. Start eating (and making) wholegrain bread, with some fresh organic fruit or vegetable, a bit of nuts, seeds, or legumes, and more rarely, a bit of dairy products or healthy meat, and then, you won't feel the hunger non-stop, but you will start losing weight.

Nutrient content of different food

The second reason you should eat more vegetable than animal food is the nutrient content of that food. As you can see in the tables below, vegetable food contains more nutrients than animal food, except some rare cases, such as Calcium in milk or vitamin A in calf liver. However, our body can absorb only a small percent of the Calcium in milk, while the vitamin A is not needed in those amounts a calf liver contains. It would be a vitamin A overdose for our body.

PROTEINS (amount (mg) per 100 g of food)			
Soy	38	Tuna	21
Sunflower seed	27	Chicken	20
Lentils	24	Veal	20
Chickpeas	23	Pork	19
Almond	18	Lamb	19
Peanuts	16	Eggs	13
Barley	14	White cheese	8

Many people claim you will not ingest enough proteins if you do not eat more meat. That is simply not true. Not only that there are more proteins in vegetable food, but the structure of animal proteins make it harder for our body to digest and absorb them. An excess of animal proteins causes health deterioration, since our body is the body of a herbivore.

VITAMIN A (amount (mg) per 100 g of food)			
Alfalfa	5300	Calf liver	6060
Carrot	4500	Tuna	970
Spinach	4300	Cod fish	939
Turnip	3000	Butter	181
Mango	1600	Cow's milk	10
Parsley	1200	Veal	6
Apricot	933		

VITAMIN B1 (amount (mg) per 100 g of food)

Wheat sprouts	2	Beef liver	0,3
Wheat	0,7	Egg yolk	0,2
Almond	0,7	Veal	0,15
Soy	0,63	Fresh salmon	0,1
Lentils	0,5	Lamb cutlets	0,1
Chickpeas	0,4	Cow's milk	0,04
Blackberry	0,3		
Pea	0,28		

VITAMIN B2 (amount (mg) per 100 g of food)

Walnuts	1	Veal	0,3
Wheat sprouts	0,8	Ham	0,2
Almond	0,6	Eggs	0,2
Avocado	0,2	Cow's milk	0,2
Peach	0,05	Tuna	0,19
		Chicken	0,17

VITAMIN B6 (amount (mg) per 100 g of food)

Wheat sprouts	4	Sardine	0,97
Walnuts	0,87	Pork	0,5
Brown rice	0,67	Veal	0,4
Soy	0,6		
Avocado	0,5		
Banana	0,37		
Pepper	0,27		
White flour	0,18		

VITAMIN C (amount (mg) per 100 g of food)

Rose hip	600	Cow's milk	2
Kiwi	300	Salmon	0,9
Alfalfa	183	Meat	0
Pepper	131	Eggs	0
Cabbage	105		
Oranges	59		
Strawberries	58		
Lemon	51		

VITAMIN E (amount (mg) per 100 g of food)

Almond	25,2	Grouper fish	0,9
Soy	13,3	Butter	2,2
Walnuts	12,3	Eggs	0,8
Sunflower seed	10	Beef liver	0,7
Wheat sprouts	8	Sheep leg	0,5
Olives	6	White chicken meat	0,3
Raspberries	4,5	Cow's milk	0,1
Pepper	3,1	Pork	0,1

VITAMIN K (amount (mg) per 100 g of food)

Turnip greens	470	Calf liver	86
Kale	360	Cheese	33
Cabbage	90	Milk	3,5
Lettuce	35		
Spinach	25		
Pea	15		

CALCIUM (amount (mg) per 100 g of food)

Sesame	783	Yellow cheese	810
Soy	260	White cheese	300
Almond	252	Cow's milk	120
Hazelnut	225	Eggs	58
Spinach	126	Salmon	14
Walnuts	87	Chicken	12
Peanuts	74	Lamb	12
Oat	70	Beef	4

IRON (amount (mg) per 100 g of food)

Soy	12	Beef liver	11
Sesame	10	Beef	3
Bean	7,6	Lamb	2
Pistachio	7,3	Pork	1,5
Lentils	7	Eggs	1,3
Sunflower seed	7	Tuna	1,2
Chickpeas	4,8	Chicken	1
Wheat	4,3	Cow's milk	0,2

MAGNESIUM (amount (mg) per 100 g of food)

Sunflower seed	420	Mutton	24
Cacao	420	Grouper fish	24
Almond	252	Hake	21,3
Soy	242	Pork	15,7
Walnuts	185	Eggs	14
Broad bean	164		
Integral flour	109		
Spinach	55		

What meat (not) to eat

Besides eating more vegetable than animal food because of its nutrient content and our body herbivore anatomy, you need to know two more things about the meat you should eat.

The first thing is that not all meat is healthy, and I am not only talking about the unhealthy aspect of too greasy and fried or dried meat; it's about the unhealthy meat of animals that are not supposed to be eaten at all. There is a simple rule to remember about avoiding this class of meat, a rule established on the basis of scientific research. This rule says: **Do not eat the meat of any animal that does not have split hooves and that does not cud its food**.

For example, you should not eat pork, because a pig, although has split hooves, yet does not cud its food. Its meat is unhealthy and inappropriate for humans to consummate. A pig and other omnivores were made to clean the ground off the corpses of dead animals. Try to avoid this meat, but if you must eat pork, it is highly recommendable to eat it in smaller amounts than before. Or as another example, you should not eat rabbit meat, because a rabbit, although cud its food, yet does not have split hooves. Its meat, too, is unhealthy and should not be eaten. Try to avoid it.

You can also put this rule in a different way, if it is easier for you to remember it: **Do not eat the meat of omnivores, predators or carnivores, and scavengers** (and some herbivores). This implies not eating a lobster, either, because it's an omnivore sea animal. And concerning fish, **you should only eat fish that has fins and scales**. For example, you should not eat catfish, because it does not have scales and it's also an omnivore sea animal (fish). The same goes for dolphin or shark meat; they do not have scales.

There is a lot of animals remaining whose meat you can freely eat: beef, veal (cattle), venison (deer), lamb, mutton (sheep), goat meat, antelope meat, moose, and so on. However, you should not eat the meat of pig (pork, bacon, ham, sausage, lard, ham…), dog, cat, horse, bear, camel, beaver, elephant, squirrel, snake, turtle, crocodile, rat, frog, crow, swallow, vulture, eagle, insects (excepting some of the locusts), and so on.

Basically, the meat of all omnivore and carnivore animals is not intended for human consumption, while the meat of the most of herbivore animals is fine. **If you eat the healthy meat, you will be healthy and lose weight, but if you eat the unhealthy meat, you will**

stay obese and get sick. It's simply the way it is, and you can't do anything about it but either obey the rule imposed by nature or break the rule and suffer the consequences.

And the second thing about eating meat concerns its production. The meat of most animals, including the healthy meat of herbivores, is often treated with too much of the toxic chemicals, additives, and taste-enhancers, just like all other food sold at stores, and besides, most of the farm animals are treated with antibiotics and other drugs, living in very harsh conditions on the farms without much sunlight and physical activity. That way, you get meat of bad quality made out of sick and drugged animals. This is why you should be careful when buying meat, and this is another reason to prefer vegetable food above meat products.

The safest thing to do is to buy meat of organically grown animals raised on pastures and fed with unprocessed food. For that reason, you should find a reliable person who knows how to farm and feed animals properly, and who produces and sells healthy meat. An alternative solution would be to have your own meat production if you live in a countryside. There is simply no other way, because almost all meat and other animal products, and almost all food sold at stores, is not healthy and directly causes obesity.

You can buy all your food from a reliable individual food producer, or at health-food stores and at the marketplace, or make your own garden and grow food you like.

The meat-tasting food without meat

Actually, there is one more solution. I could say it is a very intriguing solution that you might like. Maybe you have heard of it before, but in any case, it's probably the easiest way to replace meals with unhealthy meat as its main ingredient. Instead of that kind of meat, you can eat healthy food that has almost the same exact look and taste as regular meat, and I am not talking about taste-enhancers, such as those substances that give a meat-like taste (usually used for ham and sausage, for example), or MSG (used almost in all food products).

No, I am talking about real clean, unprocessed, chemical-free and nutrient-rich healthy vegetable food that tastes like meat. If you can't live without meat, that is, if your habit of eating meat too often is hard to quit, then you should definitely try this food. I promise you won't notice any difference, except that you won't know what kind of "meat" it is.

I remember what I thought when I ate it for the first time: We had a mixture of some vegetable and that "meat" for a lunch usually once a week, and I thought it was some kind of meat, but was not able to determine of which animal. It had a taste of meat and it looked like meat. The taste was mild, but pleasant, and the "meat" was a bit softer than the real meat, but I still couldn't get it. If nobody told me later what it was, I would have never thought it to be anything else than meat. And I bet you wouldn't guess it either, you too would think it was meat, if nobody told you what it really was. But let's not disclose the secret right away. Check what it is in the last chapter of this book where I discuss weight-loss recipes...

Wrong weight-loss diet food

Every weight-loss diet that prescribes avoiding any of the main diet ingredients – grain (bread), fruit, vegetable, legumes, and nuts – is wrong. One of the most popular "weight-loss diets" is the one forbidding you to eat cereals or grains (bread). That is ludicrous, simply said. Bread is the most important ingredient of every diet, no matter if you want to lose weight or not. If you had to pick only one food to eat for the rest of your life, in order to survive, it would have been bread. Nothing else could be compared to it, because it is the only food that could give you all nutrients necessary for survival.

Also, weight-loss diets that prescribe eating only fruit for breakfast (like an apple) are wrong, too, because a breakfast must be a large meal and must include bread besides fruit (or vegetable) and nuts. Otherwise, eating only fruit for a breakfast would cause an instant glucose (sugar) increase in your blood and then a sudden drop in its level because of the insulin production, as well as possible stomach problems.

Any diet focused on only one type of food is detrimental to your health, and all diets focused on large quantities of fat or proteins have the same effect. The foundation of your diet should be carbohydrates, but not excluding fats and proteins. Your food should be diverse and always include grain, fruit, vegetable, nuts, and legumes, because these ingredients will provide your body with all nutrients it needs.

There are also some "weight-loss diets" that prescribe eating only food that is possible to grow in your climate area. It does make sense, but this is not necessary; you can eat any food you want. The same applies to those diets prescribing eating food that is "in accordance with your blood group", which is non-sense, because your blood group has nothing to do with the food you eat.

You should not adhere to any unusual weight-loss diet, that sounds too strange or weird to you. There is a reason why it sounds that way – because it IS strange. Like I said before, there is nothing unusual and special about the ways and diet for losing weight; there are no tricks and no shortcuts. Just a bit of normal daily exercise (walking), breathing clean air, exposing to sun, eating the right food at the right time, drinking lots of water, proper resting, good mentality, and of course, body cleansing…

7. BOWEL CLEANSE

Finally, the seventh step of the program is bowel cleanse. As previously said, the cleansing program actually includes not only bowel cleanse, but also the liver cleanse and all other organs cleansing, though bowel and liver cleanse are the most important and the first to be done.

Everyone who is obese has clogged (constipated) bowels. If you relieve bowel constipation, you will quickly lose weight. How do you know if and to what extent your bowels are constipated? It's simple. Just answer this question: How many times a day/week do you empty your bowels? If it is once in 2-3 days or less frequently than that, it means your bowels are highly constipated. Even if it is once a day, it still means your bowels are constipated. The truth is that you should empty your bowels 2-3 times a day, depending on how much you eat every day. In other words, **you should empty your bowels after each meal**. If you eat a breakfast and a lunch, you should go to toilet twice a day, and if you eat a breakfast, a lunch, and a dinner, then you should go to toilet three times a day.

In order to relieve constipation, you should cleanse your bowels and eat only the food that does not cause constipation, that is, the food mentioned in the previous chapter. Avoid all other food. **All animal food, especially the processed unhealthy food sold at stores, causes constipation**. It's a fact. However, healthy food itself is not enough to thoroughly cleanse the bowels and other organs, neither any laxative will do any good, be it natural laxative herbs and food, or pharmaceutical laxatives, because those can only relieve constipation for a short period and should not be used for too long anyway; otherwise, they would cause "lazy bowels" – the incapability of emptying the bowels without taking laxatives. Coffee produces the same effect.

You need to cleanse the bowels not only with food that relieves constipation, but you also need a strong agent that will break and dilute the hardened material in your bowels, and cleanse the remaining toxins. The best method to do that is to drink **senna tea** or **herbal products based on senna**.

You can even make the senna constipation-relieving product all by yourself. You will need these ingredients: buckthorn, senna, mint, fennel, garlic, ginger, and cayenne. You will need these ingredients to be dry and grounded. Just mix all ingredients and take a teaspoon of it in water, juice or tea just before sleep. If it does not relieve constipation, increase the dosage each evening for a half of a teaspoon, until your stool softens.

Drinking enough clean water every day, an hour of daily physical activity, and a healthy diet will accelerate the process of bowel cleansing and losing weight as its consequence. Physical activity especially is great for impaired bowel movements.

Also, besides this, you can do an **enema cleanse** or a **hydro-colon therapy**. Both methods are easy to do and have a tremendously good effect on speeding your bowel movements, necessary for losing weight.

Liver cleanse

Another important organ to cleanse is the liver. It can easily be done just by drinking a juice made of these ingredients:

- 250 ml of juiced oranges and a lemon / or 250 ml of juiced apples
- 250 ml of non-carbonated water
- 1-4 cloves of garlic
- 1-4 tablespoons of olive oil
- 1 cm of ginger root

Mix all ingredients in a blender and drink the juice before the breakfast on an empty stomach.

On the first day, you should use only one clove of garlic and one tablespoon of olive oil. On the second day, take two of each; on the third day, take three of each, and on the fourth day take four of each, and then continue with four on the fifth, sixth and seventh day. So, you drink this juice for 7 days.

After that, you should drink this juice, in order to cleanse your kidneys and bladder:

- 1-2 juiced lemons
- 0.5-1 l of water
- 1/4 of teaspoon of cayenne pepper
- Honey or maple syrup

Mix all ingredients in a blender and drink the juice. Do it for the next 7 days. After that, drink the first juice again for 7 days, and then this juice for another 7 days. That is how you will cleanse the liver and other organs.

Juice fasting

A special method of body cleansing is called "juice fasting". This is not a necessary step of the program, but it is recommendable. It implies not eating any food for a short period of time, but only drinking fresh juices and water.

All you should do is **drink only water and juices you made from fresh fruit or vegetable**, as much as you want throughout the day. (It is advisable not to drink anything after 7 PM so as not to go to bathroom late at night.) Juice fasting should ideally last for at least 5 days. If you cannot take it that much, do it for less than 5 days. The longest period is 30 days.

For all that time you won't feel too much hunger, despite not taking any real food, because the juices will provide you with all nutrients your body needs for the time being, and most importantly, juices will cleanse all your organs. With bowel and liver cleanse being done at the same time, this method will tremendously accelerate the process of losing weight. Moreover, not only that you will not feel hunger, but you will gain an inexplicable amount of energy by drinking juices, since there is no digestion process occurring in the stomach when drinking the fruit and vegetable juices. For that reason, this method is also called "energy bombing".

Water fasting

It will probably sound too much for you, but whether you try the juice fasting method or not, you could also try another method, called water fasting: It consists of **not eating any food for just a single day a week** (night-day-night period).

If you abstinate from eating and drinking anything except water for just a day every week, you will not only cleanse your whole body thoroughly, not only give a proper rest to your stomach and other organs, and not only start losing weight at an incredible speed, but all your body functions and your overall physical and mental health will significantly improve, and your mind and body will be refreshed and regenerated. It is an incredible feeling of great energy, freshness and motivation. Although these two methods may sound too much for you to handle, trust me, it isn't that hard, it's all in your mind, in your way of thinking, in your desire to lose weight. It all depends on you and your wish to become healthy and fit, and to get the desired weight.

Nevertheless, if you feel you are not ready for this, you don't have to do it and push yourself to the limits. In that case, stick only to the rest of the program.

OVERVIEW – A FEW THINGS TO REMEMBER

First thing first, let me emphasize that if you cannot follow the whole weight-loss program and adhere to all its components, then you don't have to. Do as much as you can, do not overpush yourself. See what suits you the most and at what speed you can progress. Try to apply as much of the program as possible, but go slowly and gradually. There is nothing hard about it, though. You can surely do it. Even if you apply only a small part of this program, you will experience improvements very soon and you will lose weight.

So, let's make an abstract of everything said so far. I will list what you should do starting from the time you wake up until you go to bed:

1. **When you wake up, drink a glass of lukewarm water**. (It should be lukewarm, so that your stomach does not have to warm it up and lose energy right at the start of a day.)
2. If you want to, you can **take a shower in the morning, using hot and cold shower method**. (Not too cold and too hot, and not for too long. Do it gradually, using your sense of reason. Do not overpush it.) This will wake you up and increase your blood circulation – a thing very convenient for losing weight.
3. **Eat a large meal for your breakfast 1-2 hours after you get up**. It should contain wholegrain **bread, fruit, and nuts**. You can also add a dairy product if you wish to, such as yoghurt, but it is not necessary.
4. During the day, depending on your daily duties, **take a walk for a whole hour**. This physical activity part MUST NOT be avoided. Always do it. Walk every day. Spend time outdoors as much as possible, exposing your body to fresh air and sunlight.
5. Have a lunch at least 5 hours after the breakfast. It should contain wholegrain **bread, vegetable, and nuts or/and legumes**. You can also add meat if you wish to, such as veal or mutton, but it is not necessary.

6. If you have more free time, you can **read a book about health or watch a video of similar content**. Call your dear friend and **talk about good things and good people**, or reconcile with someone you offended or hated him/her for any reason. **Spend more time with your family and friends**.
7. **Go to bed before 10-11 PM with an empty stomach**. Or if you have to eat something, let it be a very light dinner at least 3.5 hours before going to bed (5:30-7 PM) and at least 5 hours after the lunch.

For the end, let us revise some of the tips for losing weight:

- **Drink at least 6-8 glasses of water a day**, preferably much more.
- **A minimum of 5 hours of pause between meals**.
- **Do not eat anything between meals**. Your stomach needs rest.
- **Do not drink anything during the meal**. It will stop digestion.
- **Do not drink anything right after the meal**.
- **Do not drink anything just before the meal**.
- **Do not drink anything except water, teas, and juices**. (No Coke, no soda, no juices from the store, no alcohol, no coffee, no energy drinks.)
- **Do not drink tap water**.
- **Always have a breakfast**. A large meal.
- **Avoid dinner**. Eat 2 times a day.
- **Be physically active for an hour a day**. A simple walking will do.
- **Spend time outdoors as much as possible**. Expose your body to fresh air and sunlight. Go to mountainous countryside occasionally.
- **Spend time with family and friends**. Do not gossip. Do not think negatively. Do not talk about anything inappropriate. Do not think only about your needs. Help others and see what their needs are.
- **Be mentally active**. Always explore and read about healthy living and ways to help others. Develop your skills and knowledge in order to do that.

- **Go to bed on time** (before 10-11 PM). Sleep in a complete dark and silence. Sleep for 6-8 hours.

If you cannot follow the whole program at the moment, then at least do these three most important things: **Drink more water** every day, **never skip a breakfast**, and **walk for about an hour** every day.

However, as you can see it yourself, I believe there is nothing hard here or too complicated, nothing that you already did not know. What did I tell you to do except things you already do, only in a bit different manner?

For example, I told you to drink water, as everyone does and must do, but I only said to **drink more water** than you usually do.

I told you to be physically active, as everyone is and should be, but I only said to **be more physically active**, and yet I didn't say you must run and jump all day, but only walk every day, as you already do, the difference being that from now on you should walk for an hour every day.

I also told you to rest, as everyone does and must do, but I only said to have a proper rest and **go to bed before 10-11 PM**.

I told you to eat food, as everyone does and must do, but I only added you should **eat the right food** and explained why that food is good for losing weight. I did not say you must eat only this or that; you can eat almost anything, but not buy that food in the stores and supermarkets. There are no strict diets and no food restrictions, but there is a sense of reason in choosing healthier food and avoiding food that contains toxins. It cannot be simpler and any more reasonable than that.

I told you to spend time on fresh air and expose your skin to sunlight, as everyone does, but I only added to **do it more often and to spend time outdoors as much as possible**, especially in the rural mountainous areas.

And finally, I told you to hang out with your friends and family, as everyone does, only adding you should do it more often and that you should try to see what other people's needs are.

Now tell me, is there anything in this program that sounds unusual or illogical to you? Is there anything complicated or hard to understand? I believe everything is clear and logical enough. **This weight-loss program practically represents the ideal way of life for every person**, even if he does not need to lose weight. Slim people who use this program will not lose weight, but will actually gain it, while obese and overweight people will lose weight using this program. In other words, the program is designed to bring everyone's weight into balance, and not only the body weight, but everything else that concerns physical and mental health.

In my opinion, this is the easiest, the most natural, and the best possible weight-loss program you will ever find. Even if you apply only a small part of the program, you will start losing weight. So, what are you waiting for? Are you ready to get your desired weight and feel younger and much more energetic? Do you believe it? Do you want it? Is there any reason why you should not try it?

Let's do it together and let's get that desired weight of yours in the shortest possible time! Let's lose some weight and live more happily! What say you?

Final Words

So, you have finally read the book, I want to congratulate you on finishing it and I hope that you use some of the information if not all.

I am giving a special script for free, these scripts contain detailed diets for anyone that wants so loose waight fast. To get these free scripts send me an email saying that you have read the book and what you think about it here: vlatkodukoski2@gmail.com and I will give you the scripts containg a secret guide that will help you lose weight even more.